DISCOVER YOUR POWER ANIMAL

NAZ AHSUN

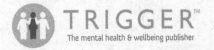

TRIGGER™
The mental health & wellbeing publisher

For the animals,
with deepest gratitude

DISCOVER YOUR POWER ANIMAL

LEARN HOW TO WORK WITH YOUR ANIMAL GUIDES

NAZ AHSUN

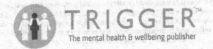

TRIGGER™
The mental health & wellbeing publisher

First published in 2021
This edition published in 2023 by Trigger Publishing
An imprint of Shaw Callaghan Ltd

UK Office
The Stanley Building
7 Pancras Square
Kings Cross
London N1C 4AG

US Office
On Point Executive Center, Inc
3030 N Rocky Point Drive W
Suite 150
Tampa, FL 33607
www.triggerhub.org

Text Copyright © 2021 Naz Ahsun

A CIP catalogue record for this book is available upon request from the British
Library
ISBN: 978-1-83796-338-6
Ebook ISBN: 978-1-83796-339-3

Cover design and illustrations by Sarah Ray at Design Marque
Typeset by Steve Williams Creative

ENDORSEMENTS

"Finally, a beautiful little book that speaks from the voice of the animals, sharing their wisdom and knowledge with us as messengers and teachers of the natural world. Overflowing with in-depth personal experience, Naz shares her unique stories of our animal helpers who choose to walk by our sides as our protectors and guardians."

Barbara Meiklejohn-Free - The Highland Seer
Bestselling and award-Winning author of *The Shaman Within*,
Shamanic Medicine Oracle Deck, *The Shamanic Handbook*.

"This little book is an easy and informative guide to help us understand and harness the magic of animal 'medicine'. It will tug at the soul of anyone who has an affinity with animals, our co-inhabitants of this planet. Naz has a natural writing style and intuitive connection to the animal kingdom and gives us a very real insight into the magical messages that the animals are trying to tell us, if we will just open our hearts and listen. Finally, the animals have their voice!"

Flavia Kate Peters - The Fairy Seer

"During these times of rampant industrialised consumerism and technological alienation, human beings have become miserably disconnected from the natural world. This book helps to reconnect. As an intuitive guide, Naz walks along-side the reader encouraging them through this wonderful soul journey of animal medicine. Full of practical tips and methods, this book will equip you with the tools you need for not only a greater connection of the many layers of self but also a deeper connection to the world soul."

Tree Carr, author of *DREAMS: How To Connect With Your Dreams To Enrich Your Life*

"I love dipping into this little book whenever I'm in need of extra inspiration. Reading *Discover Your Power Animal* is a wonderful ignition to one's own intuition."

Menna Van Praag, author

"When I look into the eyes of a gorilla, I feel a deep connection; being in their presence is therapeutic. This book has reaffirmed why I have those feelings and provoked me to delve deeper into discovering the amazing power of animals. It has shown me that the more we connect with animals and protect nature, the better off we are. A remarkable message!"

Dr. Gladys Kalema-Zikusoka, National Geographic Explorer and Founder, Conservation Through Public Health

"This is a brilliant little book, which will empower everyone who reads it with an open mind and heart. Naz Ahsun writes clearly and precisely, never preaching but always offering excellent advice. Embrace the wisdom that permeates this book, and move forward to a higher state of consciousness. I thoroughly recommend this amazing book and hope it helps and empowers every reader, as it did for me."

Kit Berry, author of the Stonewylde Series

"Oh my goodness — what a gem of a book. The inspiration to connect to your chakras and your power animals is ingenious! What insights and BIG 'ohhhh' moments I received. It truly is a book of personal and spiritual discovery. Thank you so much, Naz, for birthing this beautifully crafted and insightful book. I love it!"

Caroline Mitchell, Dragon Path Oracle Cards

CONTENTS

Chapter 3: *The Power Animal*
Wisdom Oracle   79

INTRODUCTION

Our connection to the animal kingdom has been a continuous love affair. From the earliest history of humankind, we have been dependent on the animal kingdom and nature for our very survival. When we consider the ancient society of the Mesopotamians, the Celts and the indigenous cultures of the world, such as the Salish, Apache and Lakota of North America, the Konkani people of south-western India and the Aborigines of Australia, it is clear that the interdependent relationship between humankind and nature is an ancient one.

Irrespective of our technology-filled world, our connection with and love of animals continues to thrive, whether as cat and dog lovers or through the names we use for clothing brands and cars. Even our language is immersed with animal symbolism – for example, in descriptions like 'as angry as a hornet', 'as blind as a bat', 'eager beaver', 'as free as a bird' and so on. When you begin gathering the evidence, it is astonishing really how much we still maintain our connection with the animal kingdom, irrespective of the high-speed, stress-filled ingredients that make up modern-day living.

So, is this just coincidence? Or is there something else at work – something beyond the material world and the mechanical function of our minds?

In early 2012, my life was particularly stress-filled. I was racing through my days at high speed, focused solely on my goals. I wasn't particularly satisfied with this lifestyle, as I was essentially existing from one task to the next. No surprise really that my stress levels were high and my sense of wellbeing at an all-time low.

I recall a particular Sunday evening when I was feeling especially down about my job, my home and my life in general. I felt lost, stuck in a quagmire, slowly sinking deeper and deeper. That's when I decided to call a close friend and ask her advice about how to get my life flowing again.

I don't know quite what I was expecting, but it certainly wasn't the advice she gave me, which felt like something out of Avatar! She suggested I should look for the answers through animal messengers or 'power animals', as she called them. If I slowed down, tuned into my environment and then asked the universe to send me a message through a power animal, they would appear. But how would I know if the animal was a messenger or just a random sighting, I asked. My friend assured me that I would be able to tell the difference, as the power animal would gain my attention by behaving in an unusual way. I was very dubious but, feeling I had nothing to lose, I decided to give it a go.

The next day, I felt more than a little foolish as I drove to work at half my usual speed, mentally asking the universe to send me a message through a power animal. I wondered how this would happen on a journey that mostly involved motorways. My scepticism seemed justified, as not one animal showed up, not even a gnat. By the time I got to work, my disappointment was complete. I felt beyond stupid and even lower than the night before. How gullible was I? Just as that thought crystalized, a miracle appeared.

Out of nowhere, a robin materialized and landed on my side mirror simply watching me, its burnished red breast vibrant in the morning light. My heart hammered in my chest as I stared at the robin staring, intently, back at me. Its inquisitive black eyes communicated a self-assurance and calm that I had never felt before – a feeling that all was well. It stayed there, holding my gaze, for about five minutes. Even after the robin flew off, I simply sat there, stunned by my experience.

The rest of the day passed in a haze. When I got back home, I instantly looked up what a robin power animal meant on the internet. No surprise that the robin's message was one of courage, hope, letting go of the old, viewing life from a different perspective and welcoming in new growth and opportunity.

Since that morning, a new world has opened up for me. My experience set me on a new course, where I have explored the gift of power animals in their various forms. I have developed a deep appreciation and gratitude for them and how they can support us in our day-to-day lives if we open ourselves up to hearing, seeing and feeling them.

So, I invite everyone who is reading this to join me. Simply slow down and tune in carefully to your environment so that you, too, can hear the wisdom these truly amazing animal messengers bring.

Naz Ahsun

How to Use This Book

The whole purpose of writing this book is to open a doorway to a world where you can experience your own connection with your power animals and access their insight, support and wisdom.

Please note that I use the words "power animals" as a collective term to describe all the different types of animal messengers, and I call our personal power animals "animal guides" for clarity. I share messages and guidance from 21 power animals, as well as ways for you to connect to your own animal guides, to deepen your connection and relationship with them. You'll also discover how to work with your power animals and your chakra energy system to reveal more in-depth information about you and your physical, mental, emotional and spiritual wellbeing.

This book is an introductory guide and the messages shared in it are just the tip of the iceberg. As you develop your own connection to your power animals, you may well discover that they offer you further insights and interpretations.

You can use this book in a number of ways to maximize your experience of power animals. There is no right or

wrong way to use the information provided,
so my invitation is to explore with curiosity and find
what works for you.

◈ If you begin to see an animal frequently and feel it
has a message for you, you can simply look it up in
Chapter 3: The Power Animal Wisdom Oracle (see
page 79). You will find two meanings or messages
and you will need to decide which message honestly
resonates with you. Once you have read the meaning,
you can work with the energy of that particular
power animal by reflecting on the key question and
completing the suggested activity and chakra exercise.
Each animal is linked to a particular chakra and the
chakra exercise is a simple way to utilize the energy of
the power animal to clear or energize that chakra.

◈ It is easy to use the Power Animal Wisdom Oracle
(see page 79). Simply close your eyes and ask for the
guidance you seek by thumbing through the pages of
the chapter until you feel the urge to stop. Then, read
the message from the power animal on that page.
Again, for a deeper understanding, you might wish to

reflect on the key question, or complete the activity and chakra exercise associated with that power animal.

◆ To help you connect with your own personal animal guide, I have included Your Animal Guide Meditation Journey (see page 39) to help you discover and tune in to them.

◆ To deepen your connection with the power animals, I have included a chapter on how to use your chakras (see Chapter 2: Power Animals and Your Chakra Energy System), which also contains a guided meditation (see page 75) to help you connect with your power animals.

◆ Any animal has the potential to be a power animal, so if any not in this book come into your life, do some research and try to discover why they have appeared to you by finding out which qualities they are associated with and making your own interpretations.

Chapter 1:

WHAT
OR WHO
ARE
POWER
ANIMALS?

The Universe is always communicating with us, and one way it does this is through power animals, who are healers, teachers and guides here to support us on our life journey. They are messengers from the universe who share their specific and individual gifts with us. These might manifest in a direct message from them, or they might share their natural abilities and talents; most importantly, they are here to help us realize how magnificent we are. In our ancient past, power animals were very much part of our ancestors' stories, so they do not belong to one particular group, culture or region, but to us all. However, unlike the indigenous cultures, the majority of us have forgotten this innate connection today.

There are a number of ways we unconsciously tap into the natural healing abilities of animals. For example, research shows that petting an animal reduces stress levels and anxiety, and consequently they are often used in therapy. Some institutions, such as prisons, use animals to cultivate trust, an open heart and compassion in their inmates. Some schools use dogs to support anxious young pupils and therapy pets are often firm favourites with elderly residents in care homes.

Animals have a lot to show us about being well in ourselves; they are natural healers and teachers who can guide and support us through all areas of our lives.

There are four main ways in which our natural power animals manifest.

YOUR PERSONAL ANIMAL GUIDE

Each and every one of us has our own power animal, a personal animal guide who is here to support us in our day-to-day lives. They are connected to you and, often, they are with you from birth, imbuing you with their particular gifts and abilities. They are also here to teach you more about who you are; you may discover that you have similar gifts and characteristics to them. Personal animal guides can change throughout your life, so you might find that your guide changes to offer the specific support you need as you grow older or develop and encounter new challenges and growth opportunities. However, your guide may stay with you for life. There is much you can learn from them about your gifts, talents and power.

Sometimes, they can be long-term daily companions, appearing in physical form. For example, your pet might be your animal guide in a physical guise, and if this is the case, don't be surprised if you develop a strong telepathic link.

THE MESSENGER ANIMAL

A messenger animal's role is to bring you much needed communication from the Universe and they can show up anywhere and anytime in your life in all sorts of ways. They are not usually your specific animal guide, only appearing to give you a message that you need to hear at the time, unlike your own animal guide, who is always with you. The message can be one of reassurance, warning, insight or pointing out an opportunity; in fact, the message can be anything pertaining to your life at that moment. For example, my first ever encounter with a messenger animal was with a robin, which I mention in the Introduction (see page 15). It's a message of hope, new beginnings and opportunity, which was very important for me to hear at the time, because it gave me the motivation to go in a new direction. The robin was also different from my personal animal guide because it didn't stay with me constantly, but simply appeared that one time. You might also see an animal act out of character or do something odd or significant – if so, take it as a sign that a messenger animal is communicating with you. Alternatively, you might see the animal messenger in a vision or a meditation, see the same kind of physical animal wherever you go, or hear about that particular animal in conversation. You may see pictures and images of the animal, whether on TV, the internet, a t-shirt or a poster. The point is that the animal will continue to show up until you receive their message – they can be very persistent until you do!

You can also ask the universe to communicate with you through a messenger animal, which is exactly what I did before I encountered the robin. You may like to use the Power Animal Wisdom Oracle (see page 79) to help you with this. In whatever way your messenger animal manifests themselves, rest assured that they are here to bring you useful and timely information that can help you.

THE JOURNEY ANIMAL

The journey animal is different from your personal animal guide and the messenger animal, as they travel with you into the spiritual dimensions to help you determine the best course of action, as well as teach you valuable life lessons on the journey. If you are doing a meditation, you can also choose the particular animal to journey with (see page 52) if you wish, or simply see which animal appears. Journeying involves travelling into the non-physical world and spiritual dimensions to retrieve information that will support you in the physical world. Your Chakra Meditation Journey with Power Animals (see page 75) allows you to pick the journey animal yourself, as well as the chakra you wish to explore – it's like stepping through a doorway into an element of your soul, where you discover more of your identity, your gifts and the ways you limit the ability of your soul to express itself through your physical being.

The journey animal can also appear in your dreams and take you into the dream world, sharing their message and teachings with you there. Ultimately, their purpose is to help you gain a true sense of yourself and what works for you.

They can help you find the answers that live deep within you, offering their innate wisdom and resources for you to tap into, and thereby discovering more of your own.

YOUR SHADOW ANIMAL

Your shadow animal is one of your strongest allies and greatest teachers. They are here to reveal those parts of yourself you don't like and to challenge you to be your authentic self. They are different from your personal animal guide, journey and messenger animals in that you are likely to fear or dislike them, and their sole purpose is to make you aware of those parts of yourself you have judged and rejected. You might not even be aware of how much you reject parts of yourself or self-sabotage, which is why they appear in your life. They are likely to come to you in a recurring dream or you might even have a particular phobia of them.

It is important to realize that your shadow animal isn't here to judge or punish you, but to help you integrate those aspects of yourself that you have rejected through your judgment of what is good and bad. Your shadow animal can also help you face your fears and recognize that you are a magnificent being who is capable of overcoming the challenges in your life. They might even suggest that some of these challenges could be opportunities for personal growth.

LEVELS OF COMMUNICATION WITH YOUR POWER ANIMALS

Power animals seek to communicate with you on a number of levels, including physical, mental, emotional and spiritual.

Physical

If an animal is behaving strangely, or you continue to notice a certain animal showing up frequently in your life, it is most likely there to give you a message.

Just over two years ago, I lost my pet cat, Zeus, who was my personal animal guide. Three weeks before he died, I recall curling up with him for a cuddle and feeling a wave of deep sadness and despair as I sensed that his time had come to leave me. I was close to tears and wondered how I was going to cope without him. As I sat stroking his soft, grey fur, he curled up closer to me, and then I heard a voice say very clearly inside my mind, "You have another cat coming," and I was shown an image of a sweet black-and-white kitten. Zeus lifted his head and looked at me, purring away as I continued to stroke him. I was stunned – and doubtful to say the least – as I had promised myself that I wouldn't have any more animals after him. I'd certainly had no intention of looking for another cat.

As the days ticked by, the incident kept playing on my mind and I began to see black-and-white cats everywhere, where before there had been none. The day eventually came when Zeus had to be put to sleep. I was grief-stricken after the procedure and just wanted to be left alone to mourn. However, the very same evening a friend I hadn't seen in months turned up at my home unexpectedly. She came in for a cup of tea and I told her about Zeus; she immediately mentioned that she knew of some kittens in desperate need of rescue – I felt the hairs on the back of my neck rise and I recall my exact reply, "They're black and

white, aren't they?" To say that her face was a picture is an
understatement. And when she got out her mobile phone
to show me the photos, I saw one of a sweet, black-and-
white kitten looking back at me – the very same one I had
seen in my vision.

As you can see, there are a number of ways you can
encounter an animal – it doesn't just have to be in the
flesh. I once remember seeing a swan, then an image of
a swan on a pub sign and the written word 'swan' in a
newspaper, all in one day, when swans were not creatures
I usually came across. The key is just to slow down and
become aware of your environment.

Emotional

If you have picked up this book, it is likely that you already
feel some emotional connection to the animal kingdom.
You might be a cat- or dog-lover, or simply love animals in
general. Alternatively, you might be at the other end of the
spectrum – perhaps there is a specific animal you loathe,
one that causes you to freeze in fear? If it is fear you feel,
you have most likely come into contact with your shadow

animal, hence the strong emotional response.

My own shadow animal is a snake. I used to love snakes – I even wanted a pet snake when I was in my teens, but my love soon turned to fear after recurrent dreams about a snake. In the dream I desperately try to prevent the snake from biting me. It is wrapped tightly around my right wrist and, as I wrestle with it, my fear threatens to choke me. The dream snake strikes the flesh between my thumb and forefinger, and I feel its venom burning and throbbing like fire as it penetrates my hand. To survive, I know I have to transmute the venom. Even though I can feel the panic of impending death, I know I have to remain calm for the process to work.

Now, anyone can be forgiven for wanting to forget their nightmares, but nightmares can give us huge insights into what is going on beneath the surface of everyday consciousness. In my case, my shadow animal is challenging me to be my real self. By transmuting the poison in my dream, I can move past my own personal blocks to be open, authentic and honest, speaking my truth and walking my talk, rather than worrying about others' opinions.

Your own responses toward certain animals may be varied and it is important that you pay attention to and explore them. If you have a fear or a phobia of specific animals, use it as an opportunity to explore what lies beneath this aversion – perhaps you are facing your shadow animal?

Mental

Whether you are connecting with your personal animal guide, or messenger, journey or shadow animal, you can explore its traits by doing some research. Read about the key characteristics of this creature; look up stories or legends about it; investigate the animal's habitat and what it eats and how it sleeps; and discover how it overcomes challenges; all this information can give you insights into why it has appeared in your life and how it can support you.

When you are next watching a wildlife programme, consider which animals you are drawn to and which ones repel you. Draw up a list. Do you remember which animals you liked as a child? Has that changed? All these are interesting clues you can use to determine how power animals are looking to support you now.

Spiritual

I believe that the guidance of our power animals can really help us in our day-to-day lives, as well as support us in connecting to the truth of who we are, which goes far beyond our personality. We are more than our thoughts, culture, background, social group or familial story. We are souls who have chosen to incarnate into a physical body and experience life on Earth as human beings.

Life is uncertain, and we are often presented with the unexpected. Consequently, the guidance of our power animals, who walk beside us, within us, below us and above us, is doubly important. They can help us integrate all aspects of ourselves and support our embodiment of our physicality, to truly embrace the gift of being ourselves – connecting to our true identity and who we really are.

We are continuously invited to discover how capable and brilliant we are through personal challenges, loss, success, failure, relationships – in fact, through all areas of our lives. This is where our power animals can really help us. By connecting with their energy, we can gain a greater sense of intimacy and connection with ourselves, others and the universe – an interconnected web of existence. Whatever

your query, be assured that your power animal can guide you
to the answers, which live deep inside you.

HOW TO CONNECT
WITH YOUR PERSONAL
ANIMAL GUIDE

There are many ways to connect with your personal
animal guide. Some traditional ways involve a shamanic
practitioner locating your power animal and blowing it into
your essence. However, you can also undertake the journey
yourself through Your Animal Guide Meditation Journey,
which follows (see page 39).

While on that journey, you will travel to a different
dimension, where power animals reside. There are three
dimensions, known as the lower, middle and upper worlds. We
exist in the middle world. It is a material and solid world that
we can see, hear, feel and touch and it is where we have our
primary experience as human beings. The upper world is the
realm where we connect with angels, universal consciousness,

spirit guides and other celestial beings. The lower world is where we find nature spirits and power animals. This doesn't mean that you won't find power animals in the other worlds, but their tendency is to gather in the lower world.

You might be very surprised by who your personal animal guide is, so let go of any preconceived ideas before you undertake the journey to find and connect with them. Just remember that your animal guide is the perfect ally. Once you have connected with them, it is crucial that you build a relationship and honour them – after all, they have chosen to be your ally, not the other way around. You can find more details of how to do this in Chapter 4: More Ways to Work with Your Power Animals.

You can honour them in a number of ways: keep symbols of your power animal in your home; take time to connect regularly with your animal guide; or donate your time or money to a charity or cause that supports your power animal, or wildlife in general. The choice is yours. But remember, if you neglect your animal guide, it will leave you. Some only stay with us for a short time, while others remain for life – but in all instances, honouring this unique relationship is key.

YOUR ANIMAL GUIDE MEDITATION JOURNEY

To connect with your personal animal guide, you will need to do a special meditation journey. As already mentioned (see page 26), your animal guide isn't chosen by you, but they choose you, so you might be very surprised by who they are. This is something I discovered during my own journey to connect with my animal guide. Ultimately, your guide is the one who will best serve you at that moment in time. They might have key characteristics or traits similar to your own. Alternatively, they might have different qualities that you are invited to explore. Even if they turn out to be one who doesn't appear in this book, you can explore them in ways that we have already touched upon (see page 20).

To meet your animal guide, you need to journey to the lower world – the dimension where nature spirits reside, from power animals to plant spirits and other nature energies.

To connect to the lower world to meet your personal animal guide, you need to create your own imaginary portal or entrance.

1. First, make sure the space where you are taking your journey is private (somewhere you will not be disturbed for the next half hour or so), comfortably warm and cleansed. You can cleanse your space by opening the window and ensuring it is clean and tidy. If you wish, you can also burn sage, a bay leaf or incense or use Tibetan chimes. Mentally set your intention as you cleanse the room thoroughly by stating what you are using the space for. For example, you could say, "I cleanse this space with the intention of journeying to find my animal guide." You should repeat this intention facing each direction: north, east, south and west.

2. Before you close your eyes, take careful note of the room you are in, noticing everything about it. This is important as the room acts as your anchor to the physical world and you will need to be able to visualize it to bring you back from your journey. Make sure you

have a glass of water ready for when you finish.

3. Sit with your feet connected to the ground.

4. Begin by becoming aware of your body, scanning it all from your feet up through to the crown of your head. Again, look around the room and be aware of all that is in it.

5. Now, close your eyes, take three deep breaths, inhaling through your nose. With each breath, become aware of the energy of your body and how it moves through you. On your third inhalation, focus on your breath moving down to your feet. Each time you exhale, feel yourself releasing the tensions of the day.

6. Next, imagine your feet growing roots that go down through the floor, through the foundations of the building and the ground below, then deeper through the sediment and soil until they push through the crust of the Earth, continuing to grow downward until they reach the core. Take a moment to feel the Earth's energy reaching up through the roots into your body.

7. In your mind's eye, imagine a place in nature that is untouched and appealing to you. This can be anywhere: a cave, an island, a beach, a meadow,

a mountain top, a forest – wherever seems safe and pleasant to you. Imagine this space in as much detail as you can. What can you see, hear, feel, touch and smell? Explore your surroundings, and as you explore, you notice an opening. You move toward the opening, watching it grow in size as you draw nearer. It is big enough now for you to step through, and you soon notice yourself in a tunnel, descending deep into the Earth, down into the rock and crystals, until you reach the bottom, where another opening appears before you.

8. As you step through the opening you find yourself in another natural environment – take a moment to notice what it is like. Where is it? What is the weather like? What is the temperature? What details do you notice?

9. Now begin to explore, using your senses to see, feel, hear, taste and touch.

10. As you continue to walk, you begin to sense that you are not alone. You might see a number of animals around you. Some may come and go, while others may appear more than once. When you notice the

same animal three times, you know that you are
meeting your personal animal guide.

11. Take some time to examine this animal. What kind of
animal are they? What do they look like? What colour
are they? What are they doing?

12. When you are ready, approach the animal
respectfully to communicate with them. Ask them
why they have appeared to you and wait for the
answer. You can then follow up with other questions
you might have. Ask them if they are willing to be
your guide. If they are, then thank them and hold
out your hand. As you do so, see your animal guide
shrink or transform themselves in some way, so that
their energy becomes part of your own.

13. Now, make your way back through the opening and
return along the tunnel. See yourself coming back
to where you started. Leave through the opening
and make your way back to your physical self in the
room. Feel yourself in your body by taking three
deep breaths, inhaling right down to your feet. With
each inhalation and exhalation, you are more present
in your body. Then sense yourself more present

again in the room by visualizing the details in your mind's eye. When you are ready, open your eyes. Take a moment to look around the room, again taking note of everything you see.

14. Move your toes and fingers to physically ground yourself. And when you are ready, get up and move around.

15. Take your time to drink your glass of water.

16. Make a note of your journey, who your animal guide is, what they shared with you and anything else you feel is significant about the journey. If you can, draw an image of your guide, noting colours and the environment in which you met them.

Once you know who your animal is, you can learn more about them in The Power Animal Wisdom Oracle (see page 79). If they are not listed there, you can explore them by doing some research (see page 192). It is important that you find ways to honour them and build a relationship with them, whether or not they are featured in this book. For example, you can create pieces of art depicting your animal guide, meditate on them or simply acknowledge their presence with thanks and gratitude at the end of each day.

This will help to maintain the bond.

Now that you have met with your animal guide, you can establish regular contact with them by simply visualizing their presence – they may or may not have a message for you. However, feeling their energy in and around you will help support you in challenging situations. You might want to keep a journal of your findings, meetings and messages as this can help develop the relationship between you and your animal guide.

Chapter 2:

POWER ANIMALS AND YOUR CHAKRA ENERGY SYSTEM

The chakra system we are familiar with in the western world has travelled a long way from its original home in India and the yogic Tantric traditions, both in distance, purpose and philosophy. The school of thought in the West is quite different from the ancient Tantric tradition, so much so, that they are really two different schools. In this book, we are working with the modern western chakra system and exploring how you can tune in to power animals and your chakra system to support your wellbeing.

Working with your power animals and your chakras can be a powerful journey into discovering more of who you are, accessing your natural resources and connecting to the innate wisdom you possess outside of your social programming, culture and upbringing. It can also help you discover yourself on a physical, mental, emotional and spiritual level, improve your wellbeing and even connect to consciousness itself. Your animal guide can help you explore the internal landscape of your chakras, which can also be portals to your soul.

WHAT ARE THE CHAKRAS?

The word "chakra" comes from the original Sanskrit word, *cakra*, meaning "wheel".

Chakras are energy centres that exist within and around our bodies. We are made up of energy and our physical body consists of various interconnecting energy systems. Some of these energy systems are not visible to us, so we don't tend to be aware of them. However, they are crucial to our functioning, our wellbeing and even our connection to consciousness itself. They manifest as energy fields invisible to the us, which are called auric or subtle bodies. These subtle bodies extend out from our physical body and have access points via the chakras that contain and allow vital life-energy through to support our existence. The subtle bodies include: the etheric body, which connects our physical body to the other subtle bodies; the emotional body, linked to our feelings and emotions; our mental body, linked to our thoughts and processes; the astral body, containing aspects of our personality and genes; the causal body, which links us to our personal consciousness and collective consciousness; and the soul body, which holds divine essence within us all. Our seven chakras also connect us to the roots of the Earth, like the trunk of a tree, helping us stay connected to this world and dimension. They reach all the way up toward the cosmos and the universe, like branches – we are, in effect, a bridge between the Divine and the material, physical world. Our chakras also offer us a vast amount of information about our physical, emotional, mental and spiritual health. We have many chakras within us; however, we are focusing on the seven basic chakras, which are connected to our lives and daily existence.

Your chakras are directly affected by your personal experiences, often becoming either blocked or unbalanced, so that their ability to channel life-force energy becomes compromised and you experience distress. For example, you might have periods of trauma, upset, sickness, confusion or feelings of overwhelm, as well as situations and obstacles that can cause your chakras to become unbalanced, limiting life-force energy from entering your physical body. The result of having blocked or unbalanced chakras is a lack of vitality and overall wellbeing, which is only too "normal" in modern life. It is during these periods that we can call for assistance from our animal guides to help us gain a deeper insight about what is happening to us, as well as aiding us in finding ways to resolve the issues, so we can regain a sense of wellness.

WHY WORK WITH POWER ANIMALS AND YOUR CHAKRAS?

Working with power animals and your chakras is a deeply healing and rewarding experience. We face challenges every single day of our lives, and life unfolds as it does, irrespective of our wants, desires or expectations. This can impact our sense of wellbeing, especially if things aren't going the way we want or expect. Notice how you might feel stressed or tired, or agitated when life isn't going the way you want it to or you resist what is happening. Your reaction impacts your physical, emotional, mental and spiritual wellbeing. It also affects your chakras and their ability to remain clear and open, so you can access life energy and vitality. For example, you might find that a current situation impacts your sense of safety and security, which is governed by your root chakra (see Root Chakra, page 56). In this case, you can call upon the assistance of the Ant (see page 83), who is aligned with the root chakra and can therefore provide you with the necessary insight you need to resolve the situation.

When working with your chakras, you can either choose to see which power animal shows up, or choose to work with a specific power animal that has a natural alignment to the chakra that needs clearing. If you are new to working with power animals, I recommend the latter method. See The Seven Chakras and Their Associated Power Animals on pages 55-73 for more details about the properties of each of the seven chakras and the power animals that are associated with them.

Once you have chosen the power animal (if you wish to do so) and identified the chakra you want to work with, you can prepare for Your Chakra Meditation Journey with Power Animals (see page 73). When going on the journey with your power animal, you are guided by their energy to the answers you need to help you clear the chakra. Using the Root Chakra and Ant power animal example again, the chakra meditation journey guides you into your Root Chakra with Ant power animal at your side, supporting you on your journey. Ant could guide you to explore the foundations in your life in detail and identify if these foundations are weak or too deep-rooted, or if you need to build new foundations. Ant's energy will work with you to begin to clear some of the distress you might be feeling within that chakra and so help you to gain clarity again. You might only need to take the journey once, or you might need to revisit it over a period of time, dependent on the issue you are seeking to resolve or integrate.

Undertaking a chakra meditation journey can also bring you face-to-face with aspects of your nature that you might not be aware of or that you have suppressed. Whatever you discover, this is a most powerful journey of integration and reclaiming your authentic self.

Working with your power animals and your chakra system can support you with:

- ◆ current challenges
- ◆ limiting beliefs
- ◆ accessing your natural resources
- ◆ developing new skills and talents

◆ becoming aware of beliefs and thought
  patterns that do not serve you
◆ ancestral healing
◆ personal empowerment
◆ self-care and self-love
◆ awakening

THE SEVEN CHAKRAS AND THEIR ASSOCIATED POWER ANIMALS

The seven chakras are located at specific points on our body, starting at the base of our spine and reaching up to the top of our head. Each chakra has a specific colour and purpose, providing information about aspects of ourselves and our life force.

The Root Chakra

Location: Base of the spine at the tailbone

Colour: Red

Physical: Hips, legs, lower back, genitals, feet

Emotional: Safety, security, resources, grounding, fear, anxiety, insecurity

Mental: Family values, beliefs, reality, relationship to mother

Spiritual: Manifestation, birth, ancestral line

Power Animals: Ant, Gorilla, Tortoise

The root chakra is all about the physical realm, how safe and supported we feel as we explore the material world we live in. It is concerned with survival and fulfilling the basic human needs such as food, shelter and safety. In addition, it is about manifestation, and using the root chakra energy to bring things into the physical world. How rooted we are in this reality also determines our sense of belonging. The root chakra represents our core family beliefs, and cultural and religious heritage, as well as our ancestral line – here is where it all takes root.

If you are experiencing challenges with family or your sense of safety and security, chances are your root chakra is unbalanced; you might feel it physically as well as emotionally and mentally.

This is when you can call on a power animal linked to this chakra to support you in resolving the issue. For example, you might call on Ant, who can help you learn about foundations and perseverance when starting anything new, rebuilding or strengthening your foundations in your life. Gorilla on the other hand can support you in dealing with unresolved family issues, while Tortoise invites you to slow down and not push yourself. Ultimately, power animals linked to this chakra take you on a journey to identify the root cause of your issue and lead you to the answers that can resolve them. You can find more information about Ant,

Gorilla and Tortoise on pages 83, 123 and 171 in the Power
Animal Wisdom Oracle chapter.

The Sacral Chakra

Location: Pelvis, womb

Colour: Orange

Physical: Reproductive system and sexual organs, bladder, kidneys, urinary tract

Emotional: Joy, pleasure, release, orgasm, fun

Mental: Creativity, innovation, originality

Spiritual: Wellbeing, abundance

Power Animals: Salmon, Snake, Spider

The sacral chakra is your creative centre and an invitation to tap into your creativity. It is also your feeling centre, where you are invited to feel and experience the full range of your emotions. This chakra is concerned with movement and flexibility, and your ability to dive into the river of life and allow your emotions to flow. By feeling and experiencing your emotions, you are able to release them, which helps you nurture yourself and your relationships. However, if you supress your emotions, they turn inward and affect your wellbeing. When this chakra is open you can access your creative genius, innovation and personal magic.

If you feel a lack in these areas or wish to develop your creativity and innovative thinking, then reach out to the wisdom and medicine of Salmon, Snake or Spider. While Salmon invites you to go within to unlock your many gifts, for the fire of inspiration, Snake acts as a powerful conduit that helps you discover the creative spark within you. Spider's eight legs represent the infinite abundance available from the universe, in this instance the abundance of creativity available to you. And so, Spider can take you on your own unique journey into this chakra to access that abundant creative energy that lives inside you. The journey is unique to you and you will be shown visions, given messages and prompts that are related to you, your life and current situation. However, whether it is to discover your innate gifts, regain your *joie de vivre* or develop your creativity, the power animals linked to this chakra can guide you through the gateway of the sacral chakra to your feeling, creative essence. For more information on Salmon, Snake and Spider, see pages 145, 151 and 157 respectively.

The Solar Plexus Chakra

Location: Upper part of your belly,
where your diaphragm rests

Colour: Yellow

Physical: The respiratory system and
diaphragm, digestive system, stomach, liver,

gallbladder, kidney, pancreas, adrenal glands,
spleen, the small intestine, the lower back,
the sympathetic nervous system

Emotional: Self-esteem, confidence,
assertiveness, power, pride, shame

Mental: Taking action, willpower

Spiritual: Relationship with yourself
and others, empowerment

Power Animals: Antelope, Horse, Tiger

Here lies the seat of your power – your will, your
assertiveness and your self-esteem. It is also the centre
of your core personality and ego and is what I call the
"action" chakra – where energy moves in the 3-D world.

From this place, you can direct the energy to put your ideas,
goals and plans into action, manifesting them in 3-D reality.

You are also invited to take responsibility for where you are in your life dependent on your action or inaction, your sense of empowerment or disempowerment. Remember that you are the author of your life and how you move through it is very much dependent on your sense of self and personal power.

When you are feeling confident, you might feel empowered and motivated. However, when you feel off-centre, your tendencies to procrastinate and a lack of confidence can affect your ability to manifest and take the next step. If you feel that you are indecisive and hesitate before taking action, then a journey with Antelope into your solar plexus chakra can help you find the motivational medicine you need to take the next appropriate action in your life. If you struggle with confidence and the idea of being powerful, then go on a chakra journey with Horse, who can teach you about the true meaning of power and help you uncover your own personal power. You might also want to discover your sense of adventure and, if so, Tiger is the one to show you the way. For more information on Antelope, Horse and Tiger, see pages 87, 133 and 167 respectively.

The Heart Chakra

Location: Centre of the chest

Colour: Green

Physical: Heart, circulatory system, lungs, hands, arms, back

Emotional: Love, grief, trust, compassion, vulnerability, kindness, empathy, intimacy, healthy boundaries, gratitude, self-acceptance and self-love, honesty, authenticity, jealousy, envy, forgiveness, anger, joy, grace

Mental: Sociability, openness, balance between emotions and logic

Spiritual: Interconnectedness, inner peace, integration, wholeness, humanitarianism, altruism, service, selflessness, healing

Power Animals: Deer, Panther, Swan

The heart chakra is your gateway to unconditional love and openness, and acts as a bridge from your physical body to the universe. It is also the place of self-love and self-acceptance of who you are, from which you can discover the power of being self-centred without judgment or condemnation, literally being centred in yourself. From this place of harmony, you can find yourself in direct alignment with your world and the universe.

In this state of openness, you act as a channel, receiving messages and insights from the universe and the world around you. In addition, you can access support, solutions, opportunities, love, kindness, compassion, abundance and joy, as well as taking care of yourself and others.

In a world dominated by the mind, having an open heart can be a challenge and it is no surprise that this chakra is often blocked or needs clearing, particularly when it comes to loss, self-acceptance and not judging ourselves. When you feel a lack of trust, or fear or doubt that you are loveable, then it is time to journey with the gentle energy of Deer, whose medicine can help you to reawaken your heart. And for true intimacy ("in-to-me-see"), the courage of Panther can help you discover your divine essence, whereas the grace of Swan invites you to experience the grace of acceptance. For more information about Deer, Panther and Swan, see pages 103, 137 and 161 respectively.

The Throat Chakra

Location: Neck and shoulders

Colour: Sky blue and aquamarine

Physical: Neck, throat, thyroid, lymphatic system, mouth, teeth, arms, shoulders, hands, vocal cords, breath, ears

Emotional: Truth, creativity, manifestation, congruency, manipulation, dishonesty

Mental: Communication, speech, influence, self-expression, silence

Spiritual: Inner-truth, authentic voice, connection, life

Power Animals: Dolphin, Frog, Peacock

The throat chakra concerns self-expression and communication with the world and yourself. It is the space where you can voice your experiences, your unique perspective and your truth. It is how we communicate our reality and experiences, and how we seek to connect with others. We literally breathe life into our creations through *how* we self-express, as well as *what* we self-express.

This chakra is increasingly dominating our human lives, whether it be involving speaking, writing, singing, humming, silence, music, art, our thoughts, social media or information technology. It has the power to influence, manifest and make real most directly whatever is gestating and requiring expression within us.

The gift of this chakra is also in our ability to listen and truly hear what others are communicating by keeping ourselves open to what they are saying, or how they are feeling. This can be challenging for us, as we have all grown proficient at expressing, rather than listening and developing the ability to hear someone else's viewpoint without judgment.

We all affect each other and our environment through our speech patterns. When our throat chakra is open, we express ourselves in an honest, open way. However, if we fear to give voice to what we really think or feel, then our throat chakra becomes blocked or "armoured", which stifles our natural self-expression and we become defensive and evasive. Consider what we choose to express or not to express. What do we fear? At times, silence is an even more powerful form of self-expression.

When you feel unable to express yourself, align yourself with the communicative power of Dolphin and journey with them to rediscover your gift of language. If you need to clear the air, then tapping into the cleansing energy of Frog can bring clarity and honesty to your communication. Or you might feel that you are lacking in self-expression, in which case Peacock can help you discover your unique voice. For more information about Dolphin, Frog and Peacock, go to pages 109, 119 and 141 respectively.

The Third Eye Chakra

Location: Between the eyebrows

Colour: Indigo

Physical: Eyes, frontal lobe, pineal gland, ears, nose, nervous system, pituitary gland

Emotional: Emotional intelligence, understanding

Mental: Illusion, perspective, viewpoint, focus

Spiritual: Imagination, inspiration, insight, clear-seeing, intuition, self-awareness, wisdom

Power Animals: Bat, Hawk, Wolf

The third eye chakra has most commonly been known as the psychic centre – the place where we can learn to develop our intuitive or psychic abilities. However, it is much more than that; it is the place where we begin to connect to our universal potential and the universe itself, as well as developing our insight – our ability to see within.

It is from this space and wheel of energy that we connect with our inner vision, which operates like a guide during our human journey. When our third eye is open, we can tune into the intelligence of the universe, and see clearly and discern between illusion and reality. With this chakra we are able to glimpse beyond what we know, to all that is hidden. For some, this manifests as a seeing beyond the physical world into the spirit world. Ultimately, it is the ability to go beyond the obvious and begin to gain an understanding of the multiple spectrums of colour and viewpoints between black and white.

Our third eye is also where our focus develops, as well as our ability to choose what to focus on. When our third eye is closed or "armoured", we become defensive and sometimes only focus on what we want to see. As a consequence, our vision is limited by our capacity to look at life and our world from different perspectives or viewpoints other than our own. We begin to see the world from a one-dimensional, narrow perspective based on our own experience and what we know, so we might find it difficult to understand others whose experiences are different.

During times of loss and transition, Bat can offer you support and help you get ready for a new start. The sharp eyes of Hawk, on the other hand, can teach you how to develop the focus or vision you lack in your own life, and the howl of Wolf can act as your teacher and guide in the face of the unknown. For more information about Bat, Hawk and Wolf, see pages 91, 129 and 177 respectively.

The Crown Chakra

Location: Top of the head

Colour: Deep purple

Physical: Nervous system, pineal gland,
pituitary gland, skin, cerebral cortex

Emotional: Ecstasy, wholeness,
completeness, connection

Mental: Relationship to father,
self-knowledge, true knowing

Spiritual: Consciousness, oneness,
faith and trust in the universe and soul-self,
soul, unity, enlightenment

Power Animal: Butterfly, Crow, Eagle

The crown chakra acts as your connection to the universe and the Divine. Similar to how you connect to the physical Earth through your root chakra, you can glimpse the bigger, spiritual picture through this chakra and, once it is open, become aligned with the universal energies that allow the universe to work through you in total partnership. You are part of the interconnected web of existence that links everyone and everything, and you are bigger than your physical presence, a body within a soul.

You might find all manner of synchronicities occurring in your life without you having to do anything. For example, miracles may materialise when you most need them.

However, overstimulation of this chakra can lead to issues of feeling ungrounded or unable to feel connected to reality. Staying in the moment might prove difficult, as we might time-travel to the past or future in our minds. Consequently, we never quite land or connect with our environment or others. Alternatively, armouring or being closed to new experiences can show up as cynicism, or a lack of joy, faith or trust in life and the process of life itself.

When you are feeling lost and disconnected, a journey

into this chakra with the guidance of a power animal can bring you back to yourself. You can experience the magic of transformation with Butterfly, or if you are lacking answers, go with Crow and tread the paths of the unknown to find clarity. Alternatively, you can fly on the upper thermals with Eagle, who will connect you with your eternal, ever-present self that resides outside time and space. For more information about Butterfly, Crow and Eagle, go to pages 95, 99 and 113 respectively.

Meditation Journey with Power Animals and Your Chakras

Now that you have gained some insight into the chakras, you can use the following Meditation Journey with Power Animals and Your Chakras to help you when you need to clear or unblock them.

The chakra explanations I have provided are by no means exhaustive; they only touch the surface and are based on my personal experience of them. Ultimately, it is only through your own personal journey, exploration and connection with your own energy centres that you can

73

begin to experience them for yourself, thereby developing your understanding of them.

You can use the Meditation Journey with Power Animals and Your Chakras for each chakra by setting your intention for whichever chakra you need guidance with, and selecting a power animal linked to that chakra. Remember to also visualize the colour of the chakra you are working with in the meditation.

First make sure that you are not going to be disturbed. This includes switching off your mobile phone. You can either sit upright in a chair, or lie down or sit cross-legged on the floor. It is important that you are in contact with the ground and this reality.

Before you start, set your intention regarding which chakra you would like to explore and which power animal you wish to work with. You can do this by stating out loud or in your mind something like, "I humbly call upon the support and aid of Panther as I journey into my heart chakra for clearing and illumination." Have a glass of water ready for after the journey.

1. Before you close your eyes, take careful note of the room you are in, as it will act as your anchor to the physical world when you travel into other realms. Notice all there is to see in it.

2. Once you are ready, close your eyes and take three deep breaths.

3. As your breath deepens, begin breathing into the chakra you want to work with. Do this first by identifying where it is located in your body. Next visualize its colour. And finally, begin to take your breath down into the chakra. If it is your crown or throat chakra, then you need to visualize breathing up into them.

4. As you inhale into the chakra, watch it grow bigger and bigger until it appears as a circular doorway in front of you.

5. When you are ready, step through the doorway into the world beyond.

6. What do you notice about the environment, the atmosphere?

7. As you explore, you notice signs of life, until you see the power animal you have chosen to work with

approach you. It invites you to follow.

8. Spend some time exploring this environment with your power animal, taking note of all they have to show you.

9. When your power animal has finished showing you what you need to see, they will guide you back to the entrance of the chakra.

10. Remember to give thanks for their support, then go back through the chakra doorway.

11. As you inhale, begin to visualize the chakra doorway getting smaller and the room you began your journey in becoming sharper and more focused. With each breath, watch the chakra door continue to decrease in size and the room you started in grow bigger, until the chakra door disappears.

12. Wiggle your toes and fingers before opening your eyes.

13. Take time to orientate yourself, and when ready, gently sit up and drink the glass of water, taking your time to ground yourself in the present moment.

14. Write about your experience in a journal, noting down any insights or questions that come to you.

If you have additional questions, you can always do another journey at a later date to discover the answers, or you can take time to reflect on how they apply to you in your day-to-day life.

Chapter 3:

THE POWER ANIMAL WISDOM ORACLE

In this section of the book, you can access 21 power animal messages and activities. However, before diving into this section, make sure you have done Your Animal Guide Meditation Journey (see page 39) and connected with your own personal animal guide.

You can use the oracle by asking for guidance about your issue or situation, then randomly thumbing through it until you feel the urge to stop. Alternatively, you may wish to choose a specific power animal in this chapter to explore a particular matter or circumstance you wish to resolve. Whatever you choose, remember to also set the intention that the outcome is for your highest good. You can do this by stating it out loud or in your mind and finishing with "...whatever is in my highest and best interest."

Remember that you will be presented with two messages, one being a shadow message. You will need to be really honest with yourself about which one resonates with you. There are no negative messages, simply an invitation to acknowledge what is true for you in that moment.

ANT

Key words:
Foundations, community, perseverance

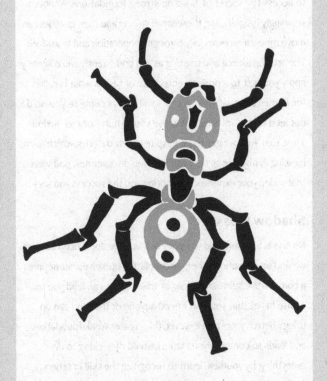

Chakra: Root

The power of patience, perseverance and persistence lies at the centre of the Ant power animal. To access Ant's wisdom is to access the secret of building strong foundations. Although seemingly insignificant, these small insects and their qualities can move mountains, especially through cooperation and teamwork. The art of patience and trusting as you consistently and diligently apply yourself to a project, enterprise or task is what is called for. Remember that what is yours will always come to you, so do not let a fear of missing out cause you to hurry or feel anxious. Trust that you can get there in spite of any detours, which are a blessing in disguise as they can help you discover new pathways that widen your experience and bring you the success you seek.

Shadow Message

No one is an island and when we act as if we don't need anyone, we end up alienating others and isolating ourselves. Sometimes a competitive spirit and a fear of missing out can lead you to a false belief that you don't need anyone or that you can do things better yourself. However, this creates weak foundations and leads to complications later. Instead of seeking to do everything by yourself, learn to recognize the skill in others, after all each person has their own special gift and talent. Teamwork is a great way of also maintaining momentum, especially when you run into obstacles. Remember, the qualities of patience and respecting boundaries are what lead to long-term, real success that you can continue to build upon.

Key Question: How do I build strong foundations?

Activity

◈ Explore how an ants' nest is constructed and look at how ants behave and work together as a team to create strong foundations.

◈ Look at the internal structure of the body and how the skeleton supports it.

Root Chakra Activity

Explore tai chi and yoga to build strong core muscles and foundations. You can get started by practising the tai chi standing postures and the yoga Downward Dog pose daily. As with any activity, do check first with your medical practitioner to ensure these exercises are suitable for you.

ANTELOPE

Key words:
Action, flexibility, attentiveness

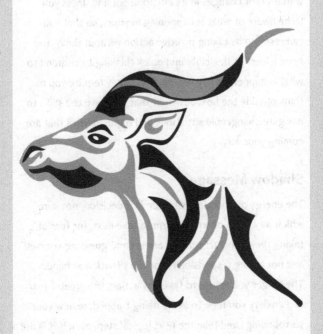

Chakra: Solar plexus

Antelope is always ready to act. Its energy is not about
standing still, but encourages moving forward. It is ever
watchful for changes in its environment and urges you
to be aware of what is happening in yours, so that you
can respond by taking positive action without delay. You
need a level of flexibility and quick thinking to respond to
what is happening in your life, which may require you to
think outside the box, but trust that you have the skills to
navigate changeable situations and opportunities that are
coming your way.

Shadow Message

The energy of Antelope is frozen in indecision, not sure
which way to go or what action to take next, for fear of
taking the wrong action. You are second-guessing yourself
and not taking responsibility for the situation at hand.
The longer you refuse to take any action, the greater fear
and anxiety you feel. To avoid being trapped, review your
surroundings and take the next logical step, even if it is not
your preference.

Key Question: What is the next appropriate action I can take in the here and now?

Activity

◆ Make a list of actions you take on a daily basis to reach your desired outcome – for example, getting to work.

◆ Change your morning routine for one month. Why not take a walk in nature or try a new route to work and notice the actions you take to navigate your way.

Solar Plexus Chakra Activity

Take up a regular yoga practice that encourages flexibility; it will open up your solar plexus and allow the energy of Antelope to connect with you. Try daily chest stretches with clasped hands behind your back. Do check first with your medical practitioner to ensure it is suitable for your level of fitness.

BAT

Key words:
Rebirth, transition, release

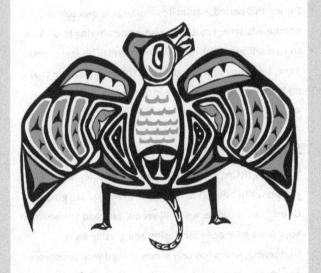

Chakra: Third eye

This is a time of rebirth and transition. What might seem like an ending is actually a new beginning, and it often involves loss. Bat energy signals that you are in the process of transformation and birthing a new aspect of yourself. During this period, Bat invites you to acknowledge and honour whatever emotions arise, remembering to be kind to yourself as you physically allow yourself to feel them. Then, be willing to let go of those things in your life that no longer serve you. You are in the process of creating space for a new period of your life to start.

Shadow Message

You are resisting progress because of your fears. Instead, you prefer to hold on to what you know. You are going through a transition, when all seems dark and unknown. Your fears have been increasing and getting more frightening, which has only strengthened your resistance and kept you trapped in your own suffering of not wanting to let go. Even though there may be a sense of loss, there is also much to be gained. Ultimately, this is a natural part of the cycle of life, which is forever moving and shifting.

Key Question: What am I ready to release in my life?

Activity

- ◈ Identify the areas in which you have felt loss and explore your feelings around this.
- ◈ Explore the cycles of the year and note down how you feel about the process of life, death and rebirth.

Third Eye Chakra Activity

Embrace silence for up to an hour each day to attune to the frequency and vibration of this chakra, which can help you connect with the place between this world and the spirit world, where Bat resides.

94

BUTTERFLY

Key words:

Abundance, transformation, new beginnings

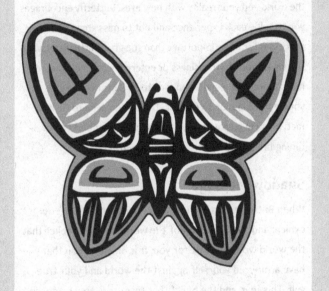

Chakra: Crown

Butterfly is a powerful symbol of transformation, heralding new beginnings and positive growth. You can be certain that new possibilities are opening up for you as you begin to see the world and your reality with new eyes. Butterfly encourages you to value each experience and not to miss steps – the process is far more important than the goal, particularly when setting up your own business or entering into a new project. It is a journey of exploration, one to be savoured, so give yourself permission to enjoy it. There is no need to rush. In fact, being in step with each unfolding moment and natural timing brings you exactly what you need.

Shadow Message

When Butterfly is stuck in its chrysalis, it points to your cynical and jaded outlook of the world and your belief that the world won't provide for you. It is an indication that you have armoured yourself against the world and your true self. This fear, and the belief that resources are scarce, cuts you off from yourself and the Universe, thus perpetuating your fears. When we are fearful, we can have a knee-jerk reaction and take foolish risks. Be mindful that now is not the time to rush ahead, but to stop what you are doing, breathe, let go of any outcomes and agendas you have and seek those who are in a position to offer you sound advice. Soon, you will begin to grow your wings again.

Key Question: How do I view new beginnings?

Activity

- ◈ Look at the metamorphosis and journey of a caterpillar into a butterfly. Journal your thoughts on this process.
- ◈ Explore the concept of birth – from the birth of the universe to the birth of a child – what do you notice?

Crown Chakra Activity

Look for signs of synchronicity occurring in your life. They can appear anywhere because the universe is always talking to you – you just have to be open to the communication. Be alert for repetitive numbers, symbols, daydreams and sudden insights.

CROW

Key words:
Omens, change, magic

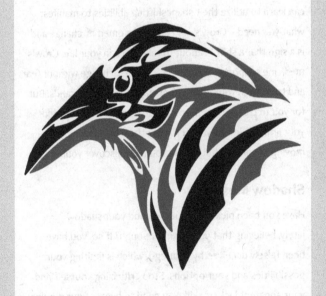

Chakra: Crown

Crow is the messenger of truth, a magician and a shapeshifter with the power of manifestation. When Crow appears in your life, you are encouraged to walk your talk and share your truth and your authentic voice. With the power of Crow, you can learn to utilize their shapeshifting abilities to manifest what you need – Crow's cry carries the omen of change and is a sign that a shift is about to take place in your life. Crow's medicine supports you in embracing that change without fear and trusting in your ability to manage the shifting sands. But for you to truly succeed, you are challenged to go beyond your limited view of yourself and others because only by moving beyond limitation can you truly discover your magic.

Shadow Message

Have you been picking at yourself and your shadow lately, believing that you are not enough? If so, you have been falsely deceived by your ego, which is limiting your possibilities and your options. Stop criticizing yourself and your apparent lack of skill. You need to bypass your monkey mind and trust your intuition. You are perfectly capable of managing whatever comes your way, but you must go deeper to connect to your truth, rather than deceiving yourself or being deceived by others about what you are truly capable of.

Your fears of the future are unfounded, as the future isn't formed yet. Remember that the future is always created in the present – and you are the author of your life.

Key Question: How does my sense of identity limit my experiences?

Activity

◈ Listen to your self-talk – how often do you criticize yourself or believe you can't do something?

◈ Draw a circle and divide it into segments representing everything you know, everything you don't know and everything you don't know that you don't know. What do you notice?

Crown Chakra Activity

Connect with your limitless self through meditation by imaging a golden light above your head, like a portal that connects you to the limitless universe. Note down your impressions.

DEER

Key words:
Gentleness, compassion, love

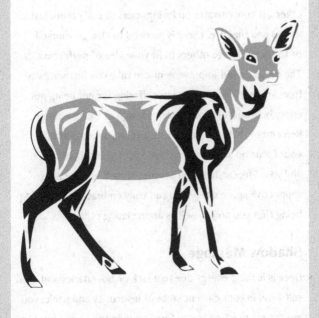

Chakra: Heart

The gentleness of Deer invites you to embrace all aspects of love and allow its energy and power to work through you. Deer is all about kindness and compassion, for yourself and others. It concentrates on loving yourself and others just as you and they are. There is no need to change yourself or to try to change others to fit your idea of perfection. The focus on self-improvement can take you further away from yourself, increasing your suffering for not being good enough, beautiful enough, slim enough or clever enough. Remember that you are perfect just as you are. Shifting your focus on all there is to love about yourself, others and your life, can help you centre yourself and create a supportive space where you can truly embrace the amazing being that you are, as well as appreciating others.

Shadow Message

Deer is leaking energy due to a lack of boundaries and self-love. In your current state of insecurity and panic, you are merely reacting to the forces moving through your life. You are reminded of the emergency airplane procedure of putting your mask on first before helping others. Nor does your willingness to play the martyr serve anyone. Instead, it creates a co-dependent relationship in which no one can realize their full potential, and long-term solutions remain out of reach. How you treat yourself is how others treat you, so if you are feeling that you are not worthy of gentleness, compassion and kindness, then others will continue to use you as a doormat. True service begins by being of service to yourself because, once you have replenished your need for kindness, compassion and love, then you will have the energy to support others who need it.

Key Question: How loving am I to myself and others?

Activity

◈ Write yourself a love letter and post it to yourself.

◈ Take regular time out to have a massage or pamper yourself, noticing the sensations this causes in your body.

◈ Monitor how you speak about yourself when you make a mistake or fail – is this similar to or different from how you speak or think about others?

Heart Chakra Activity

Go forest-bathing by spending some time immersing
yourself in the healing green colour of trees. If you live in
the city and this is not possible, introduce some potted
green plants into your home.

DOLPHIN

Key words:
Communication, play, relaxation

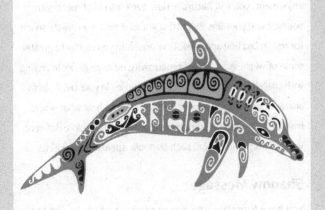

Chakra: Throat

The power of Dolphin brings you the benefits of play and fun to increase wellbeing in your life. Naturally sociable, amiable and communicative, Dolphin invites you to join the party. Through actively engaging in fun activities with no purpose other than enjoyment, you will naturally flow back into alignment with yourself and your life. By putting yourself first, you create space for rest, relaxation and work. Consequently, you can feel a greater sense of wellness, increased productivity, more resilience in dealing with challenges and also experience more joy in your life. Dolphin also asks you to develop your listening skills, to hear what others have to say from their point of view, as well as to explore different ways of communication, such as public speaking or writing.

Shadow Message

You have forgotten the power of play and all the fun has gone out of your life. Ignoring your need for self-care and relaxation leads to poor choices and less productivity, creativity and energy. Contrary to popular belief, working efficiently does not necessarily mean working extremely hard. Recognize your need to take a break and listen to your body. Dolphin urges you to come out and play and set aside the burdens you've been carrying – do not get lost in adult seriousness, as it can eventually overwhelm you. Instead, communicate your need for self-care, be honest and remember that there is so much joy to be found when you rediscover that life is for living and enjoying. Pretty soon, you'll be having fun in all areas of your life.

Key Question: How often do I take time out play?

Activity

- ◈ Take a morning out of your week to do something for fun.
- ◈ For the next month, take an hour out of your day for simple relaxation.
- ◈ Plan a fun, group activity with friends.

Throat Chakra Activity

Relax your jaw and breathe in and out through your mouth, bringing your attention to your breath as you inhale and exhale through your mouth, enjoying the sensation of simply breathing.

EAGLE

Key words:
Mastery, awareness, illumination

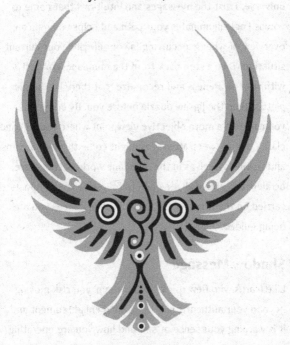

Chakra: Crown

The wings of Eagle connect you to your consciousness and awareness, soaring high into the world of spirit and the universe. Trust the messages and intuitions that come to you as Eagle illuminates your path and helps you gain an overview of what is occurring in your life and your current situation. Take a step back from the mundane, connect with your awareness and recognize that there is a bigger picture than the jigsaw puzzle before you. By doing this, you can gain a more objective viewpoint where you will find clarity and answers. Messages might come through dreams and visions as well as in the mundane world, so be aware, be alert and above all, be open to following the signposts carried on the wings of Eagle, for in all instances you are being guided.

Shadow Message

Like Icarus who flew to close to the sun, you risk moving beyond your authentic self by chasing enlightenment and it is warping your sense of self and how you are operating in the world. Be warned that Eagle's medicine is also one of cause and effect, so anything you share results in a swift response – either negative or positive depending on the authenticity behind it. Chasing enlightenment only leads you further aware from it and disconnects you from your humanity, humility and compassion. Arrogance brings a swift downfall, especially if you feel that you are superior to others and indulge in spiritual bypassing and gaslighting. Be humble and remember you are here to experience being human and it is okay not to have the answers.

Key Question: How can I take a step back when I feel confused or overwhelmed?

Activity

◈ Go to a high place – somewhere in nature like a cliff or a hilltop. If you can't access nature, then find a tall building or you can even use the first floor of your house. Now, just watch the world go by. Notice how clearly you can see when you step back to look at the bigger picture.

◈ Complete a jigsaw puzzle. Notice how the chaotic and confusing image comes together through your patient perseverance.

Crown Chakra Activity

Listen to the healing sounds from a Tibetan bowl, bell chimes or a crystal bowl attuned to the crown chakra, which can help clear and harmonize this chakra. You can listen to this on YouTube or attend a sound healing session.

FROG

Key words:
Cleansing, purification, simplicity

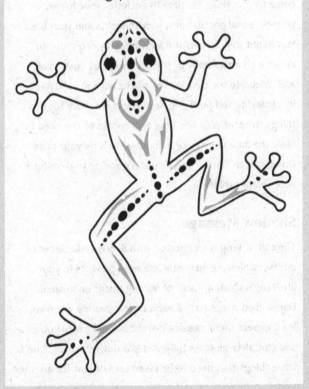

Chakra: Throat

Frog's message to you is all about simplifying your day-to-day life, your environment and your diet. If Frog has come to you, then it is time to declutter your home, your personal possessions, your thoughts and your life. You might wish to perform a giving-away ceremony to either a charity, family or friends – why not host a party and celebrate the clearing out of the old and outdated? By cleansing and purifying now, you make room for new things to enter your life. Frog also speaks of the need to clear the air and be honest about what is on your mind. Doing so can allow a deeper understanding to develop in your relationships.

Shadow Message

The call of Frog is clogged up with debris and a sense of unease, which are currently influencing events in your life. Frog's shadow warns of leaving things unfinished. Unresolved issues have a habit of reappearing when you least expect them, causing disruption. Make sure you clear and complete all tasks fully, and in a timely fashion. Don't leave things that need to be taken care of now for another

day – if you do, you risk clogging up the natural flow
of your life.

Key Question: What is no longer working for me?

Activity

◈ Make it a habit to drink plenty of water each day.
◈ Cleanse your home by opening the windows and
   allowing the purifying energy of air to blow away the
   energetic debris.

Throat Chakra Activity

Either take up singing or chant a mantra daily to clear the
stuck energy around your throat chakra.

GORILLA

Key words:
Family, ancestors, loyalty

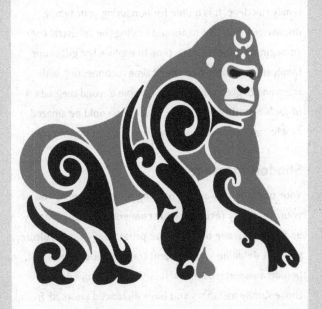

Chakra: Root

Gorilla's gentle nobility and deep links to family and
ancestors is calling you home to your family connections.
We are all inter-connected and the strong blood ties of
family run deep. It is a time for honouring your family,
discovering your forebears and healing the ancestral line.
To begin the process, take time to explore the gifts your
family have to offer you; spend time reconnecting with
them and begin to see them as people beyond their labels
of father, mother, brother or sister. You could be amazed
by what you discover and how truly fascinating they are.

Shadow Message

Your old familial ways of relating no longer serve you or
your family. By resisting your connection to your family
and the influence of your core programming and culture,
you risk deluding yourself and trapping your true spirit
behind a superficial mask. It is time to reconcile with
those family members you have distanced yourself from.
This reconciliation must be from the heart and include
forgiveness – allow them to be who they are, not who
you think they should be, so you can be who you are. It

doesn't matter if they are dead or alive or whether they wish to reconcile with you or not, it is only important that you begin healing those family wounds and stories within yourself.

Key Question: How would I describe my family in my autobiography?

Activity

❖   Make a list of positive and negative family traits and measure how long the negative list is, compared to the positive one.

❖   When with your family, focus on their positive traits rather than their negative ones. Then, see if you can add to the list of positive traits you made.

Heart Chakra Activity

Create a gratitude jar, filling it with reminders of the things you have to be grateful for. For example, you could put in a foreign coin to remind you of a holiday, a small keepsake from a relative, a flower petal from your garden, and so on. And if you don't have a physical object to add, just write down the thing you are grateful for on a piece of paper and add it to the jar. Then, whenever you are feeling a bit down, open the jar and look at your items to remind yourself to count your blessings.

HAWK

Key words:
Focus, listening, intuition

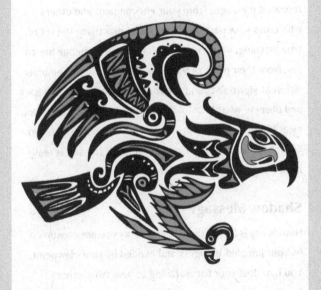

Chakra: Third eye

Listen to the whispers on the wind as Hawk carries their message to you. What needs attention? Who is asking to be heard? You will also receive further insight from repeated messages from your environment and others who cross your path. Be attentive by practising the art of true listening, where you really hear what someone has to say, from their point of view. This can help you to embrace different viewpoints and see the bigger picture. Stand back and observe what is unfolding in your life, as this gives you clear vision and the ability to access your inner sight – your "insight" – and intuition, and bring focus to what is really happening beneath the surface.

Shadow Message

Hawk's cry is lost in the wilderness, as you are consumed by your jumbled thoughts and blinded by your viewpoint. You have lost your focus, failing to hear what others have to say, because you refuse to see the situation from another perspective. You are flying blind because your ability to see the situation objectively has been seriously compromised by your unwillingness to listen to what is really being communicated. Drop your judgments and the need to be right.

Key Question: How open am I to listening to viewpoints that differ from my own?

Activity

◈ The next time you are in conversation, notice how often you mentally agree or disagree with a person, based on your own views about a subject.

◈ Try reading a book upside down, sideways, upright – which are you most comfortable with?

Third Eye Chakra Activity

Slow down and focus on the small things in your day-to-day life that you usually ignore – from waking up in the morning to buttering your toast. Note your physical sensations, your feelings and allow the Hawk's power of focus to guide you.

HORSE

Key words:
Power, empowerment, stamina

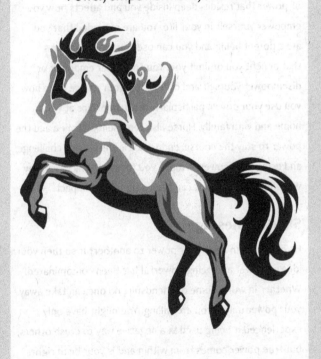

Chakra: Solar plexus

Horse speaks of true power and your ability to direct this in the real world. Horse can carry you toward your own centre of power that resides deep inside you and affects how you empower yourself in your life. You are reminded that you are a potent being and you can use your power in ways that benefit you or limit you. You can either empower or disempower yourself and others. It is your choice as to how you use your power, particularly in relationships at work, home and with family. Horse also represents stamina and the power to stay the course, endurance in the face of challenge and using your power to move you forward. Whichever way you choose to use it, it can have a significant impact.

Shadow Message

Have you given away your power to another? If so then your idea of power and being powerful has been contaminated. Whether in work, home or friendship, no one can take away your power unless you are willing. You might have only experienced it being used in a negative way to crush others, but true power comes from within and is your birth right. Rather than looking outside yourself for permission to live your life how you want to, you need to take responsibility for yourself and reclaim your ability to move forward in the direction you want to. Power can come in many forms, such as honesty, truth and authenticity, and Horse encourages you to embrace all three. Be brave and realize you have always been powerful. Do what needs to be done.

Key Question: What does power and having power mean to me?

Activity

◈ Go horse riding, if possible, and notice how the horse uses its physical power.

◈ Scan your body and note down where you feel stronger and where you lack strength. Resolve to work on the weaker parts to make them more powerful.

Solar Plexus Chakra Activity

Enjoy watching the sun rise and feel its power energizing you. Breathe in and feel its life-giving power reaching and activating your solar plexus chakra. As you exhale, image your fears dissipating.

could be like you being able to make use of talents you might be
developing and qualities in yourself. Look back, forward in the
direction you need to... kind of ... come in many forms, such as
feeling... with most animals... and make sure ... encourages you to
embrace all three... it's ... and really ... that are always here
to help you do what it means to do.

Key Question: What does power and flavor
power mean to me?

Activity

- You will need a variety of feathers and things below the heart
  chakra, physical power.
- Keep your back and butt ... how ... feel...
- She set... see about ... if ... are ... to her ... to
  and ... or parts ... or else such... are horizontal.

Solar Plexus Chakra Activity

Below you'll find some ... an exploration of the power and ... give
you freedom to... and build the inner ... breath explaining an
activity... from solar plexus chakra ... for you who has to give
your lower chakras...

136

PANTHER

Key words:
The unknown, primal, power

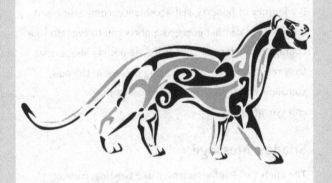

Chakra: Heart

Draw on your own courage and enter the unknown to
follow your own pathway. This is often the path less
travelled and requires your ultimate trust in the process.
The journey is of more importance than the destination,
as Panther invites you to be the authentic you, rather than
a watered-down version of yourself to please others. It
is a journey of honesty, self-acceptance, compassion and
reclamation. Panther energy supports you to tap into your
courage in the face of your fears and doubts about what
truly resonates with you. By being present in the now,
you allow the process to unfold in all its magic
and synchronicity.

Shadow Message

The energy of Panther warns of the twisting, turning
pathway built on the values of others. By pursuing this
route, you lose your sense of self and what really resonates
with you. Following the crowd might give the illusion of
safety in numbers, but it does not feed your soul nor give
you what you truly desire. Rather than run away from your
fears, you are asked to look a little deeper into them and

decide whether they are real or a figment of your fearful mind. Reconnect with your heart and reclaim what you have misplaced.

Key Question: How can I learn to tap into my courage in the face of the unknown?

Activity

- ❖ For the next five days make a list of any fears that arise during each day. At the end of the five days, identify which are current, which are old and which fears are based on the future.
- ❖ How do you feel when you drop the fears that do not apply to the here and now?

Root Chakra Activity

Spend ten minutes a day standing barefoot on the grass. Close your eyes and feel the connection between your feet and the Earth. Imagine your feet have roots that go deep down, all the way to the core of the Earth – feel her loving energy as she sustains, supports and connects you to the power of Panther.

Key Question: How can I learn to tap into / ... the ... of the unknown?

Activity

- ...
- ...

Real Chakra Activity

...

PEACOCK

Key words:
Self-expression, performance, confidence

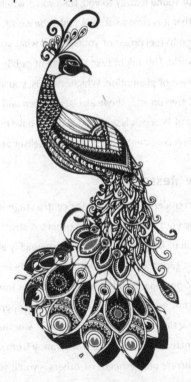

Chakra: *Throat*

Peacock energy is all about taking centre-stage and being brave enough to express and show your true colours. If Peacock has found its way to you, then you are being put on notice that it is time to step out into the world. You have every reason to feel proud of yourself and what you have to offer the world. This might take the form of public speaking, entertainment or promotion. Whichever it is, you are invited to be bold, step up and, above all else, be seen and heard. The energy of Peacock is with you and, you have every reason to feel confident in your ability to deliver and shine.

Shadow Message

Your overconfidence and desire for centre stage is threatening your relationship with others. A strutting Peacock full of hot air and no substance quickly alienates others. This superficial behaviour, where you hide behind your public persona, is only a way to hide your insecurity. You might not even be aware of how you are operating, so take the reaction of others as a clue about whether or not you are centred. Also, take your focus away from yourself and concentrate on the needs of others – you'll soon find yourself back in balance once you realize that everything doesn't always have to be about you.

Key Question: Where am I ready to shine in my life?

Activity

- ◈ Start a blog about something you are passionate about.
- ◈ Get involved in an amateur dramatic society or a public-speaking group where you can practise your self-expression.

Throat Chakra Activity

Wear bright flamboyant colours, just as the peacock displays its bright plumage, to encourage your self-expression and stimulate communication.

SALMON

Key words:
Wisdom, inner knowing, navigation

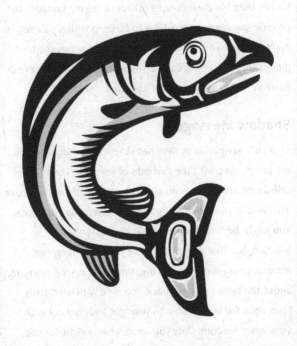

Chakra: Sacral

Salmon goes with the flow, trusting its inner knowing and inner guidance system to help it navigate the currents of life. Through inner knowing, you touch upon your own natural wisdom, even in the midst of others' judgment. Rather than blindly following others or relying on them to provide the answers, it is time to go deep within yourself and trust that your inner knowing and gut act as the best guides through any situation. You already know what needs to be done – trust your inner sonar.

Shadow Message

Salmon's navigation system has stopped working and you are out of sync with the currents of your life. The voice of self-doubt and panic is dominating your mind, and you have lost faith in your ability to navigate challenging situations. You might be tempted to opt for the easy, quick-fix solution, but that might not serve you in the long run. Instead, give yourself some breathing space, stop worrying about the future and get back into sync with what truly feels right for you – listen to your gut and connect with your inner wisdom. Only you know what is right for you.

Key Question: How often do I trust my gut and inner knowing?

Activity

◈ Connect with your inner knowing by using this visualization:

◈ Find a place where you will not be disturbed. Turn off your phone. You can sit or lie down. Take three breaths in through your nose and out through your mouth. As you exhale, release all tension and feel new energy flow in with each new in-breath.

◈ Now, follow your breath down to your gut. Really breathe into your belly, into your digestive system. Feel the area expand with each new breath; feel it awaken to new energy. How does it feel? What colour is it? Note down what you experienced in the visualization.

◈ Next time you are faced with a choice or feel confused, connect with your gut through your breath and notice how it feels.

Sacral Chakra Activity

Go for a regular swim or take a relaxing bath and feel the
energy of the water surround and support you as your
chakra opens to allow the energy of salmon through.

SNAKE

Key words:
Transmutation, healing, forgiveness

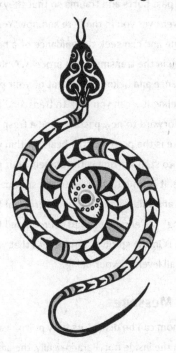

Chakra: Sacral

Snake provides healing and transformative medicine that
takes place deep within you. You are invited to shed your
old skin of past hurts and trauma so that they cease
having power over you in the here and now. You needn't
do this alone and can seek the guidance of a healer to
support you in the transmutation process. Only through
the acceptance and acknowledgment of your pain –
through feeling it – can you look to transcend the pain
and move forward to new pastures and a fresh way of
being. Snake is the power of the healer within you and
invites you to stop warring with yourself, your past and
your future. It is time to awaken to the spiritual essence of
your being and this begins with the journey of forgiveness
– "for giving" life energy back to yourself and to others
involved. It is in the spirit of forgiveness that you feel
healing on all levels of your being.

Shadow Message

Snake's venom can be deadly, its fiery poison eating those
bitten from the inside out. Paradoxically, the antidote
also lies in the venom, but requires you, the carrier, to

transmute it. So, if you have been bitten by Snake, it is likely that you are being dishonest and inauthentic in some area of your life. You might feel the effects of the poison in a physical or mental way, and it can impact all areas of your life, including your relationships. If left unattended, your dishonesty about how you really feel can keep you trapped in a cycle that will continue to bring you pain. Remember, you have the power to choose to be honest and express how you really feel, or remain trapped, stifled and in pain. You yourself are the healer you have been waiting for.

Key Question: What is ready to be healed in my life?

Activity

◈ Begin a visualized internal scan of your body. Close your eyes and start at your feet. Go within and sense the energy of your feet. Next, slowly move up to your ankles, legs and knees, then work your way up through the rest of your body until you reach the crown of your head. Notice where you feel pain (physical or emotional), then pause. Go a little deeper into the

pain, tracking it right back to the source. Notice what
happens as you take the time to really connect and
acknowledge the pain.

◈ Watch a video on how a snake sheds it skin. What
can you learn from this?

Sacral Chakra Activity

Perform a fire ceremony. Write down and express an
emotion you wish to release on a piece of paper. Light a
candle and then safely and responsibly burn the piece of
paper in the flame. Alternatively, if you are familiar with
Kundalini Shaking, you can practise this meditation for
cathartic release instead.

SPIDER

Key words:
Creativity, resourcefulness, innovation

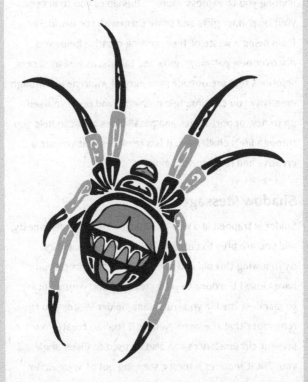

Chakra: Sacral

The artistic web of Spider encourages you to explore your own creativity, which is the universe at work within you, inviting you to express yourself. It enables you to access your own inner gifts and share them with the world. Far from being a waste of time, getting creative helps you discover new pathways, gifts and talents, as well as access solutions that are outside your current awareness. Through creativity you can untangle problems, and open yourself up to new opportunities and possibilities that can help you through life's challenges. It is a reminder that you are a creative and resourceful being.

Shadow Message

Spider is trapped in a web of entanglement and dishonesty, and you are prey to unhelpful and negative thoughts. By following this old and familiar thought pattern, you have closed the door to your creativity and your ability to manifest the life you truly want. Spider invites you to remember that the inventiveness it took to create your present circumstances can also be used to disentangle you. But it requires honesty, stepping out of your victim mindset and your habit for self-sabotage, back into the flow of inspiration. Remain patient and stay with the creative process, taking a step-by-step approach.

Key Question: How can creativity help me discover new possibilities to personal challenges?

Activity

- ◈ Cook a new meal one evening.
- ◈ Take up art, or a hobby that you have never done before.
- ◈ Explore the design of a spider's web and consider the geometry that helps it to capture its prey.

Sacral Chakra Activity

Practise moving your hips in a figure of eight motion to activate and unblock your sacral centre. Do this for up to ten minutes each day, until you feel your hips begin to loosen.

SWAN

Key words:
Grace, surrender, acceptance

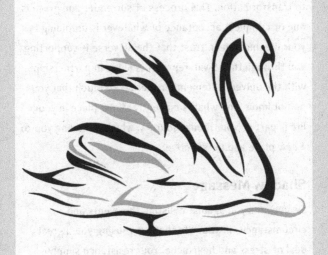

Chakra: Heart

If Swan has glided into your life, then the power of grace and surrender is at hand. By accepting and acknowledging whatever is taking place rather than resisting or seeking to control it, you open yourself up to transformation. This process of surrender and grace is one of complete acceptance of whatever is unfolding in your life and a deep trust that the universe is supporting you through this. Swan represents living in partnership with the universe. Remember there is so much that you do not know, and what is currently taking place in your life is part of your human journey, which is leading you to a new place and perspective.

Shadow Message

Swan warns you against resisting the events and circumstances in your life that are causing you a great deal of stress and heartache. Your resistance simply ensures that the external and internal conflict continues. Life may not be unfolding as you wish, but it is your reality. The sooner you stop resisting and start accepting events, the sooner you can find peace and resolution.

Life has a way of taking unexpected turns and we, as humans, feel that we have control, but this is an illusion, not a reality. The universe never sends us events we cannot deal with, but it requires us to trust in ourselves and our ability to navigate the currents of our lives when we enter rough seas.

Key Question: What am I resisting?

Activity

◈ Write ten sentences starting with "I don't like..." and complete the statement based on what is happening in your life. The longer your list, the greater your resistance to what is going on in your life. How many of the things in these statements do you have control over? What emotions are you resisting feeling? How often are you resisting the way your life is unfolding?

◈ Spend the day noticing the amount of times you or others use the phrase, "I should..." or "they should..."

Heart Chakra Activity

Dancing to tribal music with a strong beat can awaken you to the joy of being alive and the unconditional love that exists within you. Simply close your eyes and surrender to the beat of the music, allowing it to move and penetrate your heart.

TIGER

Key words:

New direction, adventure, journey

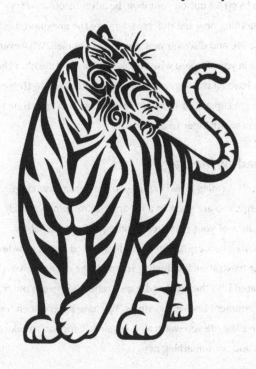

Chakra: Solar plexus

Tiger energy is all about boldly stepping into the flow of life to cultivate new direction. The power of Tiger invites you to strike out on your own, be adventurous and try something new and different. Explore the unexplored in your life and discover new aspects of yourself. Whatever area in your life you wish to take a look at, remember that you have all the resources you need within you to thrive. You are capable of more than you know. It is your time to journey with Tiger to discover it.

Shadow Message

Tiger's warning growl invites you to release your stagnant energy. You are stuck in a rut and risk isolating yourself because of your persistent limiting beliefs and habits. You are like a caged tiger prowling up and down, growling your frustration and feeling trapped. The cage you have created is in the mind and is also reflected in your outer environment and relationships. You have always been free to live the life you want; all it requires is for you to take a risk and try something new.

Key Question: What have I always wanted to explore?

Activity

◈ For one week, try something new. It could be trying a new meal, going on a different route to work or taking up a new hobby.

◈ Get a globe and write down all the countries or regions of the world you would like to visit, then consider what the next steps are to make it a reality.

Solar Plexus Chakra Activity

Include a regular exercise routine in your schedule to maintain the balance of the solar plexus and support the flow of Tiger energy through you. You may wish to take up walking or running. Do this at least three times a week.

TORTOISE

Key words:
Sacred space, grounding, retreat

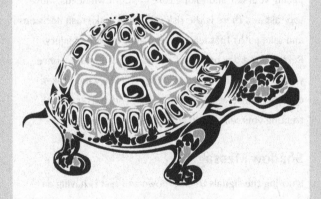

Chakra: Root

The art of grounding and slowing down is central to Tortoise's gift. You are invited to connect with the Earth, your reality, your environment and current time. Slow down and rediscover your body's natural rhythm and get back into step with yourself. This power animal is all about pacing yourself and taking care of your own needs. Move too fast and there is the risk you could make rash decisions and take paths that lead to dead ends as well as injury. Retreat for a day or two of self-care and nurture – once you remerge, all manner of things will likely have taken care of themselves. Remember that you matter – start treating yourself as you treat those you love.

Shadow Message

Ignoring the signals to slow down and rest is having an impact on your health and your lack of self-care can lead to illness and energy depletion. Tortoise reminds you of the importance of taking care of your body, as it's your home, and you are called to listen to its needs for healthy nutrition, exercise and rest. In particular, you need to find balance in your diet and include green, leafy vegetables, as well as do some gentle exercise to release the stress hormones that are currently dominating you. Contrary to popular belief, the first out of the blocks does not win the race. Life is a marathon and you, as a human, need to pace yourself and rediscover your natural rhythm – remember that life and solutions are easy to come by when you are in flow. It is you who makes it harder for yourself by rushing ahead before the road is paved.

Key Question: Do I take the time to fulfil my personal needs?

Activity

◈ Each day, take 20 minutes to simply sit quietly, doing nothing.

◈ Take your time when eating. Slow down and savour your food; really chew, smell and feel the different textures and flavours.

Root Chakra Activity

Do a walking meditation in nature, moving at half your usual pace, noticing what you see, hear, smell, feel and touch.

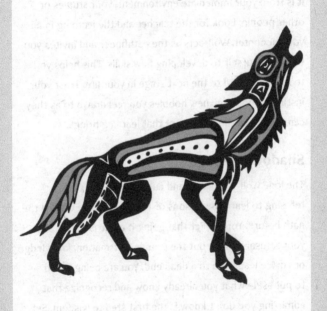

WOLF

Key words:
Instinct, learning, teacher

Chakra: Third Eye

Wolf is a powerful teacher if you are open to guidance
and wisdom. Wolf can teach you many lessons, whether
it is from your immediate environment, your studies or
other people. Look for the teacher and the learning in all
you encounter. Wolf acts as the pathfinder and invites you
to open yourself to developing new skills. This helps you
to move forward to the next stage in your life. Trust your
instincts about any new hobbies you feel drawn to as they
can teach you the enjoyment that learning brings.

Shadow Message

The lone wolf is isolated and cut off from the pack,
refusing to learn the lessons of those who have walked the
path before. Your belief that going it alone is better and
your refusal to seek out the proper information, knowledge
or advice leads you to a dead end. You are being asked
to put aside what you already know and recognize that
admitting you don't know is the first step to wisdom. Set
aside your pride and ask for help. You can always teach an
old wolf new tricks.

Key Question: How open am I to new learning and developing my skills and abilities?

Activity

◈ If you are right-handed, learn to use your left hand when writing, or brushing your teeth. Notice how easy or hard you find it. Notice how long it takes. Spend a week or two practising this new skill. How does it make you feel?

◈ Acquire a new skill that can be helpful in your job or personal life, or study something you've always wanted to learn.

Third-Eye Chakra Activity

Go moon- and star-gazing to help you connect with the wisdom of wolf and illuminate and activate your intuition – we are all part of the cosmos.

Chapter 4:

MORE WAYS
TO WORK
WITH YOUR
POWER
ANIMALS

There are a multitude of ways to work and connect with your power animals, and they are always keen to connect with you and share their wisdom. In this chapter we explore the ways in which you can do this. It is probably best to try these once you have connected with your own animal guide through Your Animal Guide Meditation Journey (see page 39).

DANCING AS A POWER ANIMAL

A wonderful and powerful way to connect with your own animal guide or any power animal and really embody its energy is through dance. This tradition was used by our ancestors to invoke the energy of a particular animal. There is no right or wrong way to do this, as it is all about the intention.

Dance has been a powerful tool for the transformation and release of energy in many cultures and has been used by indigenous culture such as the Navajo, Zulu and Maori for thousands of years. It is another way for us to experience our bodies. When we are dancing as our power animals, we really begin to feel a deeper connection with them and the wisdom they can teach us.

I once remember meeting one of my power animals in just such a fashion during an Ecstatic Awakening Dance session, which is a deeply transformational dance and active meditation. While deep in the dance, Panther came clawing out of my deepest recesses, up through my throat and roaring out of my mouth. Suddenly I was Panther and they were me, a part of myself I had repressed for years. I was so shocked by their ferocity, yet also exhilarated as I felt their energy, their primordial power. I experienced a wholeness and fierceness that I hadn't felt before. It was almost as if Panther was daring me to *be* me. That evening I accessed emotions and parts of me I had never known existed – and it was during that evening that I really felt I was coming home to myself.

You, too, can feel a closer link and gain further insight into power animals through the timeless force of dance.

1. Find somewhere private, where you won't be disturbed.
2. Set your intention and mentally invite your

personal animal guide or other power animal to dance with you.

3. Choose music with a tribal beat and when you are ready, really begin to visualize how your animal moves and mimic those movements.

4. It might feel mechanical at first, but as you continue to really embody your animal, you will find the flow. You might even end up sounding like the animal. The trick is to give your body free rein in this process, as it does not involve your programmed brain.

5. You might also feel all sorts of feelings and emotions coming through you via your animal, such as anger, freedom, sadness, joy or passion. Whatever comes through, simply allow it to be. Feel it! Dance it! Express it!

6. Your animal could bring you a message through the dance.

7. Keep up your dance for as long as you can, ideally for no less than 30 minutes.

8. Once your dance is complete, journal about your experience and remember to thank the power animal for being with you.

AUTOMATIC WRITING
AND JOURNALING

Automatic writing is an easy and fun way for you to open up an in-depth dialogue with power animals on a regular basis, or when you are stuck and need some guidance. The method is quite simple and involves the following steps.

1. Find a quiet, private space where you won't be disturbed.

2. Give yourself at least 30 minutes for this process – it might take longer.

3. Get comfortable with your paper and pen or pencil, then close your eyes.

4. Take in a few natural breaths and feel your breath fill your body. Watch it come and go. As you continue to breathe, set your intention to connect with your power animal and for them to connect with you. You might even want to ask for their assistance to help you connect.

5. With each breath begin to visualize your power animal. Do this for about five minutes or until you begin to feel their presence.

6. You can now open your eyes and begin to ask questions of your power animal by writing the question down and also noting the answer as it comes to you. Do remember that your power animals are here to help you to find solutions, not to act as oracles or fortune-tellers. Consequently, the quality of the questions you ask, determines the quality of the answers. For example, asking whether you will get your dream job, or whether the relationship you are in is right for you, may result in no response or another question. However, asking what your power animal has to share with you in your best and highest intention can lead to a more in-depth answer – you may be surprised.

It is easy to second-guess yourself when using this method, but you simply have to trust what you are writing and the answers you are being given, which can be very challenging to the logical mind. So, write what immediately comes to mind and try to ignore your monkey mind, which may try to interfere. As with most things, it gets easier with practice.

CREATING POWER ANIMAL MANDALAS

Mandalas originate from the East and are geometric designs that first appeared in Buddhism as spiritual symbols representing various aspects of the universe. They were introduced to the West through the travels of Buddhist monks who were committed to spreading Buddhism across the world.

Creating a power animal mandala can help you focus on the qualities of the power animal you wish to invoke in yourself. You can create a mandala of your personal animal guide to deepen your relationship with them, or you may wish to create a mandala for another power animal you want to connect with. This is also a great way to develop your understanding and interpretation of the power animal beyond what you have read. For example, you might create a Horse mandala for empowerment and discover more qualities of Horse than you expected by connecting with their energy.

The creation of the mandala is a meditative process and, once created, you can meditate on the mandala whenever you feel the need to connect with that power animal and evoke its energy within yourself.

INVOKING POWER ANIMALS IN YOUR DREAMS

The dream world is a powerful place where you can connect with your personal animal guide, or message, journey, or shadow animal and receive profound messages and guidance to help you in your everyday, waking life. You can also choose a specific animal to connect with because you feel drawn to them. Sometimes, they will come to you unbidden, especially if there is wisdom they urgently need to share with you; this is especially so of your shadow animal. However, you can also invoke them when you need their guidance, which requires practice and preparation.

To invoke a power animal in a dream, you can prepare in the following way.

1. Prepare an altar near where you sleep by collecting images and symbols of your power animal and placing them on it. You can also use a crystal, such as amethyst, to strengthen the connection by putting it beneath your pillow.

2. Mentally invoke the power animal you wish to

work with three times and send out an intention such as: "I humbly call upon the assistance of (the power animal you wish to work with) to meet with me in the dreaming realm and offer me guidance concerning (name the guidance you seek)." You can do this by the altar if you wish.

3. About half an hour before you go to sleep, you can also drink some "dream" tea, if you wish, such as valerian root, mugwort or blue lotus flower, but do make sure beforehand that you aren't allergic to it, and avoid mugwort if you are pregnant. These teas are perfect for evoking a lucid dream state but should only be taken at intervals and not on a nightly basis. Seek out a dream practitioner for further advice and information about dream teas.

4. Keep a journal and a pen by your bed so that you can write about your dreams when you wake up. It is best to journal as soon as you wake up, while your conscious mind is still half-asleep and you can still record the dream with accuracy.

CONCLUSION

I hope you have enjoyed this introductory guide to power animals and have managed to discover your own personal animal guide as well as other power animals and the different ways in which they manifest and operate in your life. Hopefully, you also have a better idea about working with them and your chakra energy system, as well as in various other ways, too.

The contents of this book only touch the surface of a subject that is as old as humanity. There has been much written about power animals by shamanic practitioners and shamans around the world, and let us not forget the indigenous tribes who have kept their connection to their power animal allies alive and sacred.

You can explore this topic further by browsing the internet or finding a course that will best suit you. However, nothing can really compensate for your own experience of working with power animals, nor for developing your own inner wisdom and understanding.

Wishing you a wonderful adventure,

Naz Ahsun

TriggerHub.org is one of the most elite and scientifically proven forms of mental health intervention

Trigger Publishing is the leading independent mental health and wellbeing publisher in the UK and US. Clinical and scientific research conducted by assistant professor Dr Kristin Kosyluk and her highly acclaimed team in the Department of Mental Health Law & Policy at the University of South Florida (USF), as well as complementary research by her peers across the US, has independently verified the power of lived experience as a core component in achieving mental health prosperity. Specifically, the lived experiences contained within our bibliotherapeutic books are intrinsic elements in reducing stigma, making those with poor mental health feel less alone, providing the privacy they need to heal, ensuring they know the essential steps to kick-start their own journeys to recovery, and providing hope and inspiration when they need it most.

Delivered through TriggerHub, our unique online portal and accompanying smartphone app, we make our library of bibliotherapeutic titles and other vital resources accessible to individuals and organizations anywhere, at any time and with complete privacy, a crucial element of recovery. As such, TriggerHub is the primary recommendation across the UK and US for the delivery of lived experiences.

At Trigger Publishing and TriggerHub, we proudly lead the way in making the unseen become seen. We are dedicated to humanizing mental health, breaking stigma and challenging outdated societal values to create real action and impact. Find out more about our world-leading work with lived experience and bibliotherapy via triggerhub.org, or by joining us on:

 @triggerhub_

 @triggerhub.org

 @triggerhub_

Printed in the USA
CPSIA information can be obtained
at www.ICGtesting.com
JSHW031713140824
68134JS00038B/3673